NAVIGATING PERITONEAL CANCER WITH CONFIDENCE AND CARE

Discovering Resilience And Empowering Strategies For Quick Approach And Charting Path To Cancer Healing And Holistic Wellness

DR. WESLEY IAN

DISCLAIMER

The information in this book is not meant to replace professional medical advice, diagnosis, or treatment; rather, it is meant mainly for general informational reasons. If you have any questions about a medical problem, you should always consult your doctor or another trained health expert. Don't ever discount expert medical advice or put off getting it because of something you've read in this book.

Any negative effects or repercussions arising from the usage of the material provided herein are not the responsibility of the book's author or publisher. It should be noted by readers that the material in this book is not all-inclusive and might not address every facet of the subject. Furthermore, new research may have an impact on how health concerns are understood or treated because medical knowledge is always changing.

No particular test, treatment, method, or product mentioned in this book is endorsed or promoted by the author or publisher. The reader assumes all risk associated with using the information included in this book.

Before making any big decisions regarding your health, it's crucial to speak with a licensed healthcare provider. The relationship between a patient and their healthcare practitioner should not be replaced by this book, nor is it meant to offer medical advice.

The opinions presented in this book are the author's and may not necessarily represent those of the publisher. Any errors, omissions, or inaccuracies in the information in this book are not the responsibility of the author or publisher.

It is recommended that readers independently confirm any information contained in this book and speak with a healthcare provider about their specific medical needs and state of health.

TABLE OF CONTENTS

ABOUT THE BOOK

For anyone dealing with the intricacies of peritoneal cancer, "Navigating Peritoneal Cancer with Confidence and Care" is a useful resource. The book begins with a thorough introduction that gives a general review of peritoneal cancer, clarifies its goal, and highlights the importance of confidence and care on the path ahead. This book establishes the framework for understanding and overcoming the difficulties related to peritoneal cancer, setting the tone for the entire book.

The book emphasizes a holistic approach to managing the physical, mental, and practical elements of the disease, underscoring the significance of confidence and care. The information is organized methodically and explores the different aspects of peritoneal cancer in a way that patients and their caregivers may understand.

From comprehending the nature of peritoneal cancer and its diagnostic processes to investigating treatment choices and handling the aftereffects of treatment, each component has been painstakingly created to offer a multitude of information.

Of particular interest is the book's emphasis on creating a strong support network. In addition to recognizing the critical role that friends and family play, it also explores the importance of coping mechanisms, mental health, and support groups.

To represent the most recent developments in the treatment of peritoneal cancer, this holistic approach also includes investigating treatment alternatives such as surgery, chemotherapy, immunotherapy, and clinical trial participation.

Advice on how to maintain a healthy lifestyle, balance work, and treatment, and incorporate holistic approaches into daily routines is provided by practical recommendations for daily living. In addition, the part on navigating the healthcare system offers guidance on comprehending insurance, obtaining funding, speaking up for oneself, and cultivating productive interactions with medical professionals.

With a focus on the future, the book's conclusion discusses survivability and life after treatment. It negotiates the nuances of life following therapy, clarifying the significance of monitoring, follow-up care, and accepting a new normal. "Navigating Peritoneal Cancer with Confidence and Care" is a valuable resource that provides information, encouragement, and a detailed road map for anyone dealing with peritoneal cancer.

CHAPTER ONE
INTRODUCTION TO PERITONEAL CANCER

The peritoneum, the thin layer of tissue that lines the abdominal cavity and covers the majority of the abdominal organs, is the site of origin of peritoneal cancer, an uncommon and frequently aggressive kind of cancer. The hallmark of this kind of cancer is the unchecked proliferation of cells in the peritoneum, which can result in tumors that threaten neighboring tissues and organs. Ovarian and peritoneal cancers are closely associated, with comparable symptoms, risk factors, and treatment modalities. Even though peritoneal cancer is not very frequent, early detection and efficient management depend on knowledge of the disease's features, risk factors, and current treatments.

The peritoneum is a protective membrane that is essential to the nourishment and support of the organs in the abdomen. When cancer cells grow within this tissue, they have the potential to interfere with organ function and cause a variety of symptoms, such as bloating, abdominal pain, altered bowel habits, and unexplained weight loss. Diagnosing peritoneal cancer can be difficult because its symptoms overlap with other abdominal illnesses. This emphasizes the significance of a thorough medical evaluation and diagnostic testing.

A vital component in the setting of peritoneal cancer is care and confidence. It's crucial for those receiving a diagnosis to have faith in their treatment plan and the medical staff. Positivity is nurtured by confidence, enabling patients to take an active role in their care and make knowledgeable choices. It is important to foster self-assurance in the patient to help them through the difficult process of navigating cancer treatment, in addition to fostering trust in the medical staff.

The provision of both medical and emotional care is essential to the comprehensive therapy of peritoneal cancer. Healthcare professionals must work together in a coordinated manner to implement the multidisciplinary strategy that includes surgery, chemotherapy, and other therapeutic procedures.

Furthermore, it is important to recognize the importance of patients' emotional health because receiving a cancer diagnosis can present serious psychological and emotional difficulties. The entire care plan is around giving patients a comforting setting that attends to their emotional requirements.

Peritoneal cancer is a complicated medical issue that necessitates a full comprehension of its causes, manifestations, and available treatment options. To receive complete care that addresses both physical and emotional aspects, patients must have trust in the medical staff and themselves. These are critical components in the diagnosis and treatment of peritoneal cancer. To guarantee the best potential outcomes for those impacted by peritoneal cancer, a comprehensive and patient-centered approach is still crucial as continuous research advances our understanding of this illness.

CHAPTER TWO

COMPREHENDING COLORECTAL CANCER

The peritoneum—the thin layer of tissue that surrounds the abdomen and envelops the organs—is the site of origin of peritoneal carcinoma, an uncommon but deadly kind of cancer.

The peritoneum is an essential structure that supports shields and aids in the movement of the abdominal organs. Peritoneal cancer is caused by the development of malignant cells within this tissue and is frequently identified as an ovarian cancer subtype.

Although the exact origins of peritoneal cancer are unknown, several risk factors may make the disease more likely to occur. An increased risk is linked to genetic factors, such as mutations in the BRCA1 or BRCA2 genes.

Peritoneal cancer susceptibility may also be influenced by a personal or family history of colorectal, breast, or ovarian cancer. Another important consideration is age since the danger rises with age.

Because there are no distinct signs in the early stages of the disease, it might be difficult to diagnose peritoneal cancer. However, bloating, changes in bowel habits, unexplained weight loss, and abdominal pain or discomfort are other common signs.

Given the potential for these symptoms to mimic those of other disorders, a comprehensive examination by a medical practitioner may be necessary for early discovery. This evaluation may include imaging tests, blood testing, and, in certain situations, exploratory surgery.

Depending on the cells that give rise to it, there are many forms of peritoneal cancer. The most prevalent kind, epithelial peritoneal carcinoma, arises from the cells that line the peritoneum. Primary peritoneal serous carcinoma is another kind that resembles ovarian cancer quite a bit.

A less common subtype is stromal tumors, which originate from connective tissue within the peritoneum.

The process of staging peritoneal cancer entails figuring out how far the cancer has gone; Stage I represents a limited presence, whereas Stage IV denotes extensive dissemination to distant organs.

In most cases, surgery, chemotherapy, and occasionally targeted medicines are used to treat peritoneal cancer. To remove as much of the malignant tissue as feasible, surgery may involve removing parts of the peritoneum, the fallopian tubes, the uterus, and the ovaries. Following surgery, chemotherapy is frequently used to target any cancer cells that may still be present and stop recurrence.

Peritoneal cancer is a complicated and comparatively uncommon type of cancer that affects the tissue lining the belly, or peritoneum. Although the precise causes are yet unknown, age and genetics are important predictors of the condition.

The lack of particular symptoms can make early detection difficult, but a combination of imaging tests, blood testing, and surgical exploration can help make the diagnosis. Treatment for peritoneal cancer varies depending on the kind and stage of the disease; generally, surgery and chemotherapy are used in conjunction. To effectively manage peritoneal cancer, a comprehensive and individualized approach is needed to address its distinct characteristics and problems.

CHAPTER THREE

IDENTIFICATION AND MEDICAL EVALUATIONS

DIAGNOSTIC PROCEDURES

Diagnostic procedures are crucial elements of the medical evaluation process that help medical practitioners determine the underlying reasons for a patient's symptoms or ailment. These processes cover a broad spectrum of methods, from straightforward physical examinations to more complex laboratory testing. Through scrutiny of the patient's body, palpation of certain areas, and auscultation, physical examinations enable medical professionals to obtain vital information about the patient's general health as well as any possible problems.

Important diagnostic instruments and laboratory tests offer both quantitative and qualitative information on many facets of a patient's physiology. Clinicians are assisted in assessing organ function, identifying anomalies in biochemical indicators, and detecting infections using blood tests, urine analysis, and other laboratory examinations. These tests play a crucial role in assessing the efficacy of therapies, helping to confirm or rule out particular medical disorders, and directing treatment decisions.

Improvements in medical imaging and scanning technology have completely changed the diagnostic landscape by making it possible for medical practitioners to see structures and pinpoint anomalies with unprecedented accuracy. Ionizing radiation is used in X-rays, a traditional imaging method, to create finely detailed images of bones and some soft tissues. Compared to traditional X-rays, computed tomography (CT) scans provide a more detailed view of the body by creating cross-sectional images through the use of computer processing and X-ray technologies.

Strong magnets and radio waves are used in magnetic resonance imaging (MRI) to produce finely detailed images of organs and tissues. For the examination of soft tissues such as the brain, spinal cord, and joints, MRI is especially useful. Another non-invasive imaging technique that uses sound waves to provide real-time images of interior structures is ultrasound. It is frequently used to evaluate organs like the liver and kidneys as well as to image the fetus during pregnancy.

Utilizing radioactive tracers, nuclear medicine generates images of organ function and identifies problems at the molecular level. Nuclear medicine procedures such as single-photon emission computed tomography (SPECT) and positron emission tomography (PET) scans offer important insights into ailments like neurological disorders, cancer, and cardiovascular problems.

MEDICAL CONSULTATIONS AND SECOND OPINIONS

Medical consultations are essential exchanges between patients and medical specialists since they offer a chance to go into great detail regarding symptoms, medical background, and possible course of therapy. During these meetings, good communication between the patient and the healthcare professional is essential because it promotes collaborative decision-making and helps to develop a thorough understanding of the patient's situation.

Getting a second opinion is wise in some situations, particularly when dealing with complicated or life-threatening medical issues. Seeking a second opinion from a trained healthcare practitioner entails getting their viewpoint on the diagnosis and available treatments. By doing this, you may increase the precision of the diagnosis, guarantee that the suggested course of treatment is suitable, and provide patients with more assurance when making healthcare decisions. When there is a question regarding the best course of action, vital diagnoses, or significant surgeries, second views are very valuable.

Medical consultations, imaging and scanning technologies and diagnostic procedures are all essential components of the medical assessment process. Together, these elements aid in the precise diagnosis of medical disorders, direct medical practitioners in creating efficient treatment regimens, and support patients in making educated decisions.

CHAPTER FOUR

ESTABLISHING A NETWORK OF SUPPORT

THE IMPORTANCE OF FRIENDS AND FAMILY

Creating a strong support network is crucial for overcoming obstacles and apprehensions in life. A fundamental element of this method is the resolute assistance offered by loved ones and friends. In difficult times, the importance of intimate bonds cannot be emphasized. Family members provide a special fusion of practical, financial, and emotional support because of their innate ties.

People can express their weaknesses in a secure atmosphere without worrying about being judged because of the familial relationship. Friends are selected partners on life's journey who bring different viewpoints, a range of ideas, and a sense of camaraderie that often strengthens ties to family.

NETWORKS AND SUPPORT GROUPS

Support groups and networks, which extend outside one's social circle, are essential for promoting a feeling of acceptance and comprehension. These organizations bring people together who are dealing with comparable issues, fostering a community of understanding and support. Whether coping with health problems, bereavement, or other life stresses, being a part of a support group offers a forum for sharing experiences and validation. These networks' ability to build community and resilience in the face of personal adversity is what gives them their overall strength.

COPING MECHANISMS AND MENTAL HEALTH

It is impossible to overstate the importance of mental health in the setting of a support network. Overall health is based on mental well-being, and coping mechanisms are essential for keeping things in balance. One of the proactive steps in promoting mental health is seeking professional assistance, such as counseling or therapy. Furthermore, incorporating self-care activities such as stress management and mindfulness helps improve coping skills. Acknowledging the value of mental health not only helps people deal with obstacles more skillfully but also makes the support system as a whole more resilient.

Individual and group coping mechanisms are the foundation of a strong support network. Building a toolkit of coping techniques that are specific to one's needs and preferences is essential on a personal level. This could be working out, finding artistic outlets, or doing enjoyable things. In addition, encouraging candid communication within the support network is a key component of collective coping strategies. Promoting conversations about struggles and victories fosters a culture where everyone is respected and feels heard. Common coping strategies may surface, fortifying the connections within the support network and augmenting its comprehensive efficacy.

Creating a support system is a multimodal strategy that incorporates the long-term help of friends and family, the group dynamic of support groups, and the importance of mental health and coping mechanisms. People can build a strong support network that can withstand life's inevitable storms by realizing how these ideas are interconnected. The strength of these relationships, whether it be via the love of family, the companionship of friends, or the common experiences of a support group, enables people to overcome obstacles with grace and resiliency.

CHAPTER FIVE

OPTIONS FOR TREATMENT

Peritoneal carcinoma is a rare type of cancer that affects the lining of the abdominal cavity. Surgery is a crucial part of the treatment for this disease. Often, the main objective of surgical intervention—a process called cytoreductive surgery—is to remove as much of the malignant tissue as possible. To accomplish effective debulking, this complex procedure entails excising tumors from the peritoneum and nearby organs. Additionally, surgeons can carry out operations like peritonectomy, which entails the removal of the afflicted organs and peritoneal lining. Hyperthermic intraperitoneal chemotherapy, or TIPEC, is sometimes administered after surgery to target any cancer cells that may still be present and enhance treatment results.

CHEMOTHERAPY PROTOCOLS

Whether used alone or in conjunction with surgery, chemotherapy is an essential part of the systemic treatment of peritoneal cancer. Chemotherapy regimens vary in their targeting of cancer cells and their ability to proliferate. Medications including carboplatin, paclitaxel, and cisplatin are frequently utilized. Depending on the exact treatment plan, these drugs may be injected intravenously or directly into the abdominal cavity.

Chemotherapy tries to kill all cancer cells in the body, lowering the possibility of a relapse and raising the chances of survival. Chemotherapy regimen selection is based on the specific diagnosis of each patient, taking into account variables such as cancer type, stage, and general health.

ADVANCES IN IMMUNOTHERAPY

Immunotherapy is a novel technique for treating cancer by using the body's immune system to identify and eliminate cancer cells. Immunotherapy strengthens the body's defenses against cancer; whereas conventional treatments like surgery and chemotherapy concentrate on directly attacking the disease.

Research on the use of immunotherapeutic drugs to strengthen the immune system's defenses against cancer cells in the peritoneal cavity is still ongoing in the setting of peritoneal cancer. Immunotherapy advances that are showing promise in the treatment landscape include adoptive cell therapies, immune checkpoint inhibitors, and monoclonal antibodies. These treatments provide new paths for better outcomes and fewer adverse effects.

NEW TREATMENTS AND CLINICAL TRIALS

Clinical trials play a critical role in improving our knowledge of and ability to treat peritoneal cancer. These clinical trials investigate new treatments and combinations of treatments, frequently utilizing state-of-the-art methods and technologies.

Targeted therapies that directly address the molecular features of peritoneal cancer may be among the emerging treatments; this could result in more focused and efficient interventions. Patients who take part in clinical trials may have access to novel therapies that are not yet generally available.

Ongoing clinical studies support the development of treatment approaches as scientists learn more about the complexities of peritoneal cancer, giving those afflicted by this difficult disease hope for an improved prognosis and quality of life.

CHAPTER SIX
CONTROLLING ADVERSE REACTIONS
NAUSEA AND WEARINESS

During and after medical treatments, it's crucial to manage side effects like nausea and weariness to ensure a patient's well-being. Severe nausea, frequently brought on by radiation, chemotherapy, or specific drugs, can seriously lower a patient's quality of life. To treat this symptom, anti-nausea drugs, dietary changes, and mindfulness exercises are frequently used. Comprehending the causes and trends of nausea enables medical professionals to customize treatments to meet the specific requirements of each patient, resulting in a more individualized and efficient method of managing symptoms.

A multimodal approach is necessary to address fatigue, a common side effect of many medical therapies. It's crucial to strike a balance between physical exercise and rest, as well as to eat healthily and stay hydrated. To help people become more self-aware and enable them to assess their energy levels and make wise judgments about their daily activities, patient education is essential. Integrative methods that address the mental and physical components of this prevalent side effect, such as yoga or mindfulness exercises, may also help to mitigate weariness.

PAIN MANAGEMENT

Managing pain correctly is essential to improving the general health of people receiving medical care or living with long-term illnesses. A thorough pain management strategy combines non-pharmacological and pharmacological treatments. The type and intensity of pain are major factors in the prescription of analgesic drugs, which can range from over-the-counter alternatives to opioids on prescription. To address the psychological and emotional elements of pain, a holistic approach incorporates physical therapy, acupuncture, cognitive-behavioral therapy, and relaxation techniques.

Personalized pain management programs strive to maximize pain treatment while avoiding potential adverse effects by taking into consideration each patient's particular traits and preferences. To make necessary adjustments to treatment programs and guarantee that pain management techniques fit the patient's goals and lifestyle, regular communication between patients and healthcare providers is crucial.

EMOTIONAL AND PSYCHOLOGICAL IMPACT

Patients may have significant emotional and psychological adverse effects from medical therapies. During treatment, common reactions that may surface are anxiety, depression, and feelings of isolation. To address these issues, incorporating mental health assistance into the entire care plan is crucial. Counseling, support groups, and mindfulness-based therapies are a few examples of psychosocial interventions that provide helpful tools for handling emotional distress.

By establishing a secure space where patients can voice their worries and anxieties, healthcare professionals play a critical role in encouraging open conversation regarding the emotional elements of sickness. In addition to enhancing mental health, identifying and managing the psychological implications of side effects also improves treatment outcomes overall and increases patient satisfaction.

NUTRITIONAL ASPECTS

During medical treatments, nutritional aspects are crucial for preventing side effects and enhancing general health. Appetite changes, taste changes, and trouble swallowing are frequent issues that patients may experience that affect how much food they consume. Creating a customized nutrition plan with the assistance of a trained dietitian can help fulfill nutritional needs and lessen the negative impacts of treatment-related side effects.

It is crucial to guarantee that the body receives sufficient amounts of vital nutrients, vitamins, and minerals to aid in its healing and recuperation. When eating becomes difficult, methods like dietary supplements or altered textures could be investigated.

CHAPTER SEVEN

USEFUL ADVICE FOR EVERYDAY LIFE

MANAGING TREATMENT AND WORK

Managing one's well-being requires striking a balance between employment and treatment. It's critical to discuss openly the difficulties you may have with employers and coworkers when addressing health concerns. C

Creating a positive work atmosphere can have a big impact on your general physical and emotional well-being. If at all possible, try to arrange for remote work or flexible work hours to accommodate treatment and medical schedules.

Furthermore, managing time becomes crucial while balancing obligations to one's health and career. To prevent feeling overburdened, prioritize your work, establish reasonable goals, and assign as needed. Acknowledge your boundaries and speak clearly when changes are required. Establishing a regimented schedule can help with stress reduction, control maintenance, and making sure that treatment and work get the attention they need.

SUSTAINING AN INVIGORATING LIFESTYLE

The cornerstone of total well-being is a healthy lifestyle, which includes mental, emotional, and physical health. Exercise regularly is essential for improving mood, lowering stress levels, and promoting cardiovascular health.

It doesn't have to be hard; you can make it more sustainable by choosing something you want to do, like yoga, cycling, or walking.

Another essential element of a healthy lifestyle is nutrition. Make eating a healthy, well-balanced diet high in whole grains, lean meats, and veggies a priority. Maintaining proper hydration is equally vital since it promotes healthy physical processes and mental clarity. Reducing processed food, sugar-filled beverages, and overindulgence in caffeine can have a good effect on general health and energy levels.

Although it's frequently overlooked, getting enough sleep is essential to preserving good health. Create a relaxing evening ritual, stick to a regular sleep schedule, and make sure your sleeping environment is restful. Good sleep improves immune system performance, emotional stability, and cognitive function.

INCLUDING HOLISTIC METHODS

Holistic approaches to health take into account how the mind, body, and spirit are all intertwined. Including holistic activities in daily life can improve general health and support conventional medical care. For example, practicing mindfulness and meditation can promote serenity, lower stress levels, and enhance mental clarity. These routines can be easily integrated into everyday activities, like working breaks or the time before bed.

Examining complementary and alternative therapies like massage or acupuncture may open up new possibilities for overall well-being. To make sure that these procedures complement your overall treatment plan, speak with medical professionals. A holistic feeling of wellness is enhanced by partaking in joyful and fulfilling activities, such as interacting with loved ones, exploring creative hobbies, or spending time in nature.

Furthermore, developing thankfulness and a positive outlook can have a significant impact on mental and emotional well-being. Even in difficult circumstances, finding joy in life's little pleasures can help build resilience and increase life satisfaction in general. Keep in mind that complementing holistic therapies is useful and that developing a customized strategy that takes into accounts each patient's unique needs and preferences requires close collaboration with healthcare specialists.

HOW TO USE THE HEALTHCARE SYSTEM AND RECOGNIZE FINANCIAL AID AND INSURANCE

To guarantee that people can receive the care they require without having to shoulder excessive financial burdens, navigating the healthcare system requires a critical grasp of insurance and financial aid. When it comes to paying for medical costs, health insurance is essential for both routine checkups and unplanned crises. People must understand all aspects of their insurance policies, such as coverage limitations, co-payments, deductibles, and any exclusions. With this information, patients may make well-informed decisions regarding their care and steer clear of unforeseen out-of-pocket costs.

Programs for financial help are vital resources for those in difficult financial situations. People with low incomes can frequently receive aid from hospitals and healthcare providers. It is essential to comprehend the prerequisites and the application procedure for these kinds of programs.

Further support can be obtained by looking into non-profit organizations, community resources, and government assistance programs. Financial counselors can assist people in navigating the complicated world of healthcare expenditures so they can get the care they need without jeopardizing their financial security.

TAKING UP YOUR DEFENSE IN MEDICAL SETTINGS

People must be proactive health advocates to navigate the healthcare system effectively. This entails being aware of available treatments, asking relevant questions, and actively engaging in decision-making processes. To get the best results, forming a partnership with healthcare providers is essential. Patients ought to have the confidence to express their concerns, ask questions, and give their opinions on treatment options.

People should be equipped with relevant information about their medical history, present symptoms, and any drugs they are taking to advocate effectively. Maintaining a personal health record can help with comprehensive treatment and enable more seamless contact with medical professionals. Getting second views while making important medical decisions can also yield insightful information and help create a more comprehensive picture of the range of available treatments.

When a patient is unhappy with their care, they should not be afraid to speak out for their rights and let their doctor know. A collaborative relationship between patients and healthcare providers is fostered by open communication, which eventually results in more effective and individualized healthcare experiences.

EFFECTIVE COMMUNICATION WITH HEALTHCARE PROFESSIONALS

Having good and transparent communication with medical professionals is essential to getting high-quality care. Accurate communication of symptoms, concerns, and medical history is essential for patients to help healthcare providers make well-informed decisions about diagnosis and treatment. Just as crucial is active listening, during which patients pay close attention to what their healthcare team is saying and ask questions when necessary.

People must inquire about potential drug side effects, treatment options, and health issues. By working together, the patient-provider relationship is improved and mutual trust and understanding are fostered.

Patients should not be afraid to ask for information in plain language when presented with complex medical information to ensure understanding.

Patients and healthcare professionals can communicate more easily over time by using digital communication tools like encrypted messaging platforms and patient portals. These tools offer a practical means of exchanging non-urgent information, posing queries, and getting prompt answers.

Successfully navigating the healthcare system necessitates a thorough comprehension of financial aid, insurance, self-advocacy, and effective communication. People can take charge of their healthcare journey by actively participating in these areas, guaranteeing access to high-quality care and encouraging favorable health outcomes.

CHAPTER EIGHT
LIVING AND GOING BEYOND
AFTER TREATMENT LIFE

Beyond Survivorship presents a complex journey that goes beyond the conclusion of cancer treatment. The period following treatment is crucial for helping survivors overcome the obstacles of reintegrating into their regular lives. The psychological and physical toll that cancer treatment takes frequently has a lifelong effect, forcing survivors to acclimate to a new normal. Reclaiming one's life entails dealing with the psychological and emotional fallout from the cancer experience in addition to treating the residual physical symptoms.

MONITORING AND AFTERCARE

Monitoring and follow-up care are essential to life after treatment. It becomes imperative to have regular check-ups with a doctor to watch for any indications of recurrence or side effects after therapy. These consultations act as a link between the intensive nature of active therapy and the recently attained freedom of survivorship. Healthcare professionals are essential in helping survivors get through this stage, providing support, and taking care of any new health issues. Maintaining physical and mental well-being becomes dependent upon survivors and medical experts working together.

ACCEPTING THE NEW NORMAL

One of the most important aspects of the survivorship journey is accepting a new normal. The process entails reevaluating one's goals and identity in light of the changes cancer has brought about in a person's life. It necessitates developing resilience and adjusting to a post-cancer self that integrates the pre-cancer self. Many survivors see the experience as a chance for personal development that increases their feeling of gratitude and helps them to have a greater appreciation for life. Accepting a new normal is a dynamic, ever-evolving experience that is characterized by both successes and setbacks. It is not a linear process.

Survivorship is a complex emotional landscape that includes a range of responses like gratitude, dread of recurrence, and the need for ongoing care. Participating in support groups and establishing connections with other survivors helps foster a feeling of belonging and understanding.

Dealing with the effects on relationships—whether they be with friends, family, or coworkers—is another aspect of survival. As cancer survivors and their loved ones learn to manage the altering dynamics that frequently accompany life after cancer, communication becomes essential in navigating these relationships.

Finally, a holistic journey that goes beyond the medical components of cancer treatment is embodied by survivorship and beyond. After treatment, life entails adjusting to a new normal, where monitoring and follow-up care are essential to preserving health and well-being.